Keto Diet Tracker For Faster Results And Success
(90-Days Log Book)

All rights reserved. No part of this book may be reproduced in any form by any electronic or mechanical means including photocopying, recording, or information storage and retrieval without permission in writing from the author.

Printed by CreateSpace, An Amazon.com Company

Before Keto

paste your photo here

After Keto

paste your photo here

.... Day.....................Month......................Year

M T W T F S Sun
☐ ☐ ☐ ☐ ☐ ☐ ☐

BREAKFAST

Food Item	Serving Size	Carbs	Fats	Protein	Calories

LUNCH

Food Item	Serving Size	Carbs	Fats	Protein	Calories

DINNER

Food Item	Serving Size	Carbs	Fats	Protein	Calories

SNACK

Food Item	Serving Size	Carbs	Fats	Protein	Protein

Total For The Day		Carbs	Fats	Protein	Calories

Glasses of Water:	**Comments**
☐ ☐ ☐ ☐ ☐ ☐ ☐ ☐ ☐ ☐ ☐ ☐	
Supplement Intake: Yes: ☐ No: ☐	
Electrolyte Intake: Yes: ☐ No: ☐	
In Ketosis: Yes: ☐ No: ☐	
Exercise: Yes: ☐ No: ☐	

.... Day......................Month......................Year

M T W T F S Sun
☐ ☐ ☐ ☐ ☐ ☐ ☐

BREAKFAST

Food Item	Serving Size	Carbs	Fats	Protein	Calories

LUNCH

Food Item	Serving Size	Carbs	Fats	Protein	Calories

DINNER

Food Item	Serving Size	Carbs	Fats	Protein	Calories

SNACK

Food Item	Serving Size	Carbs	Fats	Protein	Protein

		Carbs	Fats	Protein	Calories
Total For The Day					

Glasses of Water:
☐ ☐ ☐ ☐ ☐ ☐ ☐ ☐ ☐ ☐ ☐ ☐ ☐

Supplement Intake: Yes: ☐ No: ☐

Electrolyte Intake: Yes: ☐ No: ☐

In Ketosis: Yes: ☐ No: ☐

Exercise: Yes: ☐ No: ☐

Comments

.... Day.....................Month.......................Year

M T W T F S Sun
□ □ □ □ □ □ □

BREAKFAST

Food Item	Serving Size	Carbs	Fats	Protein	Calories

LUNCH

Food Item	Serving Size	Carbs	Fats	Protein	Calories

DINNER

Food Item	Serving Size	Carbs	Fats	Protein	Calories

SNACK

Food Item	Serving Size	Carbs	Fats	Protein	Protein

		Carbs	Fats	Protein	Calories
Total For The Day					

Glasses of Water:

□ □ □ □ □ □ □ □ □ □ □ □ □

				Comments
Supplement Intake:	Yes: □	No: □		
Electrolyte Intake:	Yes: □	No: □		
In Ketosis:	Yes: □	No: □		
Exercise:	Yes: □	No: □		

.... Day.................Month.................Year

M T W T F S Sun
☐ ☐ ☐ ☐ ☐ ☐ ☐

BREAKFAST

Food Item	Serving Size	Carbs	Fats	Protein	Calories

LUNCH

Food Item	Serving Size	Carbs	Fats	Protein	Calories

DINNER

Food Item	Serving Size	Carbs	Fats	Protein	Calories

SNACK

Food Item	Serving Size	Carbs	Fats	Protein	Protein

		Carbs	Fats	Protein	Calories
Total For The Day					

Glasses of Water:

☐ ☐ ☐ ☐ ☐ ☐ ☐ ☐ ☐ ☐ ☐ ☐ ☐

Comments

Supplement Intake:	Yes: ☐	No: ☐
Electrolyte Intake:	Yes: ☐	No: ☐
In Ketosis:	Yes: ☐	No: ☐
Exercise:	Yes: ☐	No: ☐

.... Day.....................Month.....................Year

M T W T F S Sun
☐ ☐ ☐ ☐ ☐ ☐ ☐

BREAKFAST

Food Item	Serving Size	Carbs	Fats	Protein	Calories

LUNCH

Food Item	Serving Size	Carbs	Fats	Protein	Calories

DINNER

Food Item	Serving Size	Carbs	Fats	Protein	Calories

SNACK

Food Item	Serving Size	Carbs	Fats	Protein	Protein

		Carbs	Fats	Protein	Calories
Total For The Day					

Glasses of Water:	Comments
☐ ☐ ☐ ☐ ☐ ☐ ☐ ☐ ☐ ☐ ☐ ☐ ☐	

Supplement Intake:	Yes: ☐	No: ☐	
Electrolyte Intake:	Yes: ☐	No: ☐	
In Ketosis:	Yes: ☐	No: ☐	
Exercise:	Yes: ☐	No: ☐	

.... Day.....................Month.....................Year

M T W T F S Sun
☐ ☐ ☐ ☐ ☐ ☐ ☐

BREAKFAST

Food Item	Serving Size	Carbs	Fats	Protein	Calories

LUNCH

Food Item	Serving Size	Carbs	Fats	Protein	Calories

DINNER

Food Item	Serving Size	Carbs	Fats	Protein	Calories

SNACK

Food Item	Serving Size	Carbs	Fats	Protein	Protein

		Carbs	Fats	Protein	Calories
Total For The Day					

Glasses of Water:
☐ ☐ ☐ ☐ ☐ ☐ ☐ ☐ ☐ ☐ ☐ ☐ ☐

			Comments
Supplement Intake:	Yes: ☐	No: ☐	
Electrolyte Intake:	Yes: ☐	No: ☐	
In Ketosis:	Yes: ☐	No: ☐	
Exercise:	Yes: ☐	No: ☐	

.... Day............Month............Year

M T W T F S Sun
□ □ □ □ □ □ □

BREAKFAST

Food Item	Serving Size	Carbs	Fats	Protein	Calories

LUNCH

Food Item	Serving Size	Carbs	Fats	Protein	Calories

DINNER

Food Item	Serving Size	Carbs	Fats	Protein	Calories

SNACK

Food Item	Serving Size	Carbs	Fats	Protein	Protein

Total For The Day		Carbs	Fats	Protein	Calories

Glasses of Water:

□ □ □ □ □ □ □ □ □ □ □ □ □ □

			Comments
Supplement Intake:	Yes: ☐	No: ☐	
Electrolyte Intake:	Yes: ☐	No: ☐	
In Ketosis:	Yes: ☐	No: ☐	
Exercise:	Yes: ☐	No: ☐	

.... Day.....................Month.....................Year

M T W T F S Sun
☐ ☐ ☐ ☐ ☐ ☐ ☐

BREAKFAST

Food Item	Serving Size	Carbs	Fats	Protein	Calories

LUNCH

Food Item	Serving Size	Carbs	Fats	Protein	Calories

DINNER

Food Item	Serving Size	Carbs	Fats	Protein	Calories

SNACK

Food Item	Serving Size	Carbs	Fats	Protein	Protein

		Carbs	Fats	Protein	Calories
Total For The Day					

Glasses of Water:

☐ ☐ ☐ ☐ ☐ ☐ ☐ ☐ ☐ ☐ ☐ ☐ ☐

Supplement Intake:	Yes: ☐	No: ☐
Electrolyte Intake:	Yes: ☐	No: ☐
In Ketosis:	Yes: ☐	No: ☐
Exercise:	Yes: ☐	No: ☐

Comments

.... Day.....................Month.....................Year

M T W T F S Sun
☐ ☐ ☐ ☐ ☐ ☐ ☐

BREAKFAST

Food Item	Serving Size	Carbs	Fats	Protein	Calories

LUNCH

Food Item	Serving Size	Carbs	Fats	Protein	Calories

DINNER

Food Item	Serving Size	Carbs	Fats	Protein	Calories

SNACK

Food Item	Serving Size	Carbs	Fats	Protein	Protein

		Carbs	Fats	Protein	Calories
Total For The Day					

Glasses of Water:	Comments
☐ ☐ ☐ ☐ ☐ ☐ ☐ ☐ ☐ ☐ ☐ ☐ ☐	
Supplement Intake: Yes: ☐ No: ☐	
Electrolyte Intake: Yes: ☐ No: ☐	
In Ketosis: Yes: ☐ No: ☐	
Exercise: Yes: ☐ No: ☐	

.... Day........................Month........................Year

M T W T F S Sun
☐ ☐ ☐ ☐ ☐ ☐ ☐

BREAKFAST

Food Item	Serving Size	Carbs	Fats	Protein	Calories

LUNCH

Food Item	Serving Size	Carbs	Fats	Protein	Calories

DINNER

Food Item	Serving Size	Carbs	Fats	Protein	Calories

SNACK

Food Item	Serving Size	Carbs	Fats	Protein	Protein

Total For The Day		Carbs	Fats	Protein	Calories

Glasses of Water:	Comments
☐ ☐ ☐ ☐ ☐ ☐ ☐ ☐ ☐ ☐ ☐ ☐ ☐ ☐	

Supplement Intake:	Yes: ☐	No: ☐
Electrolyte Intake:	Yes: ☐	No: ☐
In Ketosis:	Yes: ☐	No: ☐
Exercise:	Yes: ☐	No: ☐

.... Day......................Month......................Year

M T W T F S Sun
☐ ☐ ☐ ☐ ☐ ☐ ☐

BREAKFAST

Food Item	Serving Size	Carbs	Fats	Protein	Calories

LUNCH

Food Item	Serving Size	Carbs	Fats	Protein	Calories

DINNER

Food Item	Serving Size	Carbs	Fats	Protein	Calories

SNACK

Food Item	Serving Size	Carbs	Fats	Protein	Protein

		Carbs	Fats	Protein	Calories
Total For The Day					

Glasses of Water:	Comments
☐ ☐ ☐ ☐ ☐ ☐ ☐ ☐ ☐ ☐ ☐ ☐ ☐ ☐	

Supplement Intake:	Yes: ☐	No: ☐	
Electrolyte Intake:	Yes: ☐	No: ☐	
In Ketosis:	Yes: ☐	No: ☐	
Exercise:	Yes: ☐	No: ☐	

.... Day..................Month..................Year

M T W T F S Sun
☐ ☐ ☐ ☐ ☐ ☐ ☐

BREAKFAST

Food Item	Serving Size	Carbs	Fats	Protein	Calories

LUNCH

Food Item	Serving Size	Carbs	Fats	Protein	Calories

DINNER

Food Item	Serving Size	Carbs	Fats	Protein	Calories

SNACK

Food Item	Serving Size	Carbs	Fats	Protein	Protein

Total For The Day		Carbs	Fats	Protein	Calories

Glasses of Water:

☐ ☐ ☐ ☐ ☐ ☐ ☐ ☐ ☐ ☐ ☐ ☐ ☐

Comments

Supplement Intake:	Yes: ☐	No: ☐
Electrolyte Intake:	Yes: ☐	No: ☐
In Ketosis:	Yes: ☐	No: ☐
Exercise:	Yes: ☐	No: ☐

.... Day.....................Month......................Year

M T W T F S Sun
☐ ☐ ☐ ☐ ☐ ☐ ☐

BREAKFAST

Food Item	Serving Size	Carbs	Fats	Protein	Calories

LUNCH

Food Item	Serving Size	Carbs	Fats	Protein	Calories

DINNER

Food Item	Serving Size	Carbs	Fats	Protein	Calories

SNACK

Food Item	Serving Size	Carbs	Fats	Protein	Protein

		Carbs	Fats	Protein	Calories
Total For The Day					

Glasses of Water:	Comments
☐ ☐ ☐ ☐ ☐ ☐ ☐ ☐ ☐ ☐ ☐ ☐	

Supplement Intake:	Yes: ☐	No: ☐	
Electrolyte Intake:	Yes: ☐	No: ☐	
In Ketosis:	Yes: ☐	No: ☐	
Exercise:	Yes: ☐	No: ☐	

.... Day.....................Month......................Year

M T W T F S Sun
☐ ☐ ☐ ☐ ☐ ☐ ☐

BREAKFAST

Food Item	Serving Size	Carbs	Fats	Protein	Calories

LUNCH

Food Item	Serving Size	Carbs	Fats	Protein	Calories

DINNER

Food Item	Serving Size	Carbs	Fats	Protein	Calories

SNACK

Food Item	Serving Size	Carbs	Fats	Protein	Protein

		Carbs	Fats	Protein	Calories
Total For The Day					

Glasses of Water:

☐ ☐ ☐ ☐ ☐ ☐ ☐ ☐ ☐ ☐ ☐ ☐ ☐

Comments

Supplement Intake:	Yes: ☐	No: ☐
Electrolyte Intake:	Yes: ☐	No: ☐
In Ketosis:	Yes: ☐	No: ☐
Exercise:	Yes: ☐	No: ☐

.... Day.....................Month......................Year

M T W T F S Sun
☐ ☐ ☐ ☐ ☐ ☐ ☐

BREAKFAST

Food Item	Serving Size	Carbs	Fats	Protein	Calories

LUNCH

Food Item	Serving Size	Carbs	Fats	Protein	Calories

DINNER

Food Item	Serving Size	Carbs	Fats	Protein	Calories

SNACK

Food Item	Serving Size	Carbs	Fats	Protein	Protein

		Carbs	Fats	Protein	Calories
Total For The Day					

Glasses of Water:	Comments
☐ ☐ ☐ ☐ ☐ ☐ ☐ ☐ ☐ ☐ ☐ ☐ ☐	

Supplement Intake:	Yes: ☐	No: ☐	
Electrolyte Intake:	Yes: ☐	No: ☐	
In Ketosis:	Yes: ☐	No: ☐	
Exercise:	Yes: ☐	No: ☐	

.... Day......................Month.......................Year

M T W T F S Sun
☐ ☐ ☐ ☐ ☐ ☐ ☐

BREAKFAST

Food Item	Serving Size	Carbs	Fats	Protein	Calories

LUNCH

Food Item	Serving Size	Carbs	Fats	Protein	Calories

DINNER

Food Item	Serving Size	Carbs	Fats	Protein	Calories

SNACK

Food Item	Serving Size	Carbs	Fats	Protein	Protein

		Carbs	Fats	Protein	Calories
Total For The Day					

Glasses of Water:	Comments
☐ ☐ ☐ ☐ ☐ ☐ ☐ ☐ ☐ ☐ ☐ ☐	

Supplement Intake:	Yes: ☐	No: ☐	
Electrolyte Intake:	Yes: ☐	No: ☐	
In Ketosis:	Yes: ☐	No: ☐	
Exercise:	Yes: ☐	No: ☐	

.... Day.....................Month.....................Year

M T W T F S Sun
☐ ☐ ☐ ☐ ☐ ☐ ☐

BREAKFAST

Food Item	Serving Size	Carbs	Fats	Protein	Calories

LUNCH

Food Item	Serving Size	Carbs	Fats	Protein	Calories

DINNER

Food Item	Serving Size	Carbs	Fats	Protein	Calories

SNACK

Food Item	Serving Size	Carbs	Fats	Protein	Protein

		Carbs	Fats	Protein	Calories
Total For The Day					

Glasses of Water:	Comments
☐ ☐ ☐ ☐ ☐ ☐ ☐ ☐ ☐ ☐ ☐ ☐ ☐	
Supplement Intake: Yes: ☐ No: ☐	
Electrolyte Intake: Yes: ☐ No: ☐	
In Ketosis: Yes: ☐ No: ☐	
Exercise: Yes: ☐ No: ☐	

.... Day.....................Month.......................Year

M T W T F S Sun
☐ ☐ ☐ ☐ ☐ ☐ ☐

BREAKFAST

Food Item	Serving Size	Carbs	Fats	Protein	Calories

LUNCH

Food Item	Serving Size	Carbs	Fats	Protein	Calories

DINNER

Food Item	Serving Size	Carbs	Fats	Protein	Calories

SNACK

Food Item	Serving Size	Carbs	Fats	Protein	Protein

		Carbs	Fats	Protein	Calories
Total For The Day					

Glasses of Water:	Comments
☐ ☐ ☐ ☐ ☐ ☐ ☐ ☐ ☐ ☐ ☐ ☐ ☐	

Supplement Intake:	Yes: ☐	No: ☐	
Electrolyte Intake:	Yes: ☐	No: ☐	
In Ketosis:	Yes: ☐	No: ☐	
Exercise:	Yes: ☐	No: ☐	

.... Day..................... Month..................... Year

M T W T F S Sun
☐ ☐ ☐ ☐ ☐ ☐ ☐

BREAKFAST

Food Item	Serving Size	Carbs	Fats	Protein	Calories

LUNCH

Food Item	Serving Size	Carbs	Fats	Protein	Calories

DINNER

Food Item	Serving Size	Carbs	Fats	Protein	Calories

SNACK

Food Item	Serving Size	Carbs	Fats	Protein	Protein

Total For The Day		Carbs	Fats	Protein	Calories

Glasses of Water:	Comments
☐ ☐ ☐ ☐ ☐ ☐ ☐ ☐ ☐ ☐ ☐ ☐ ☐	

Supplement Intake:	Yes: ☐	No: ☐	
Electrolyte Intake:	Yes: ☐	No: ☐	
In Ketosis:	Yes: ☐	No: ☐	
Exercise:	Yes: ☐	No: ☐	

.... Day.....................Month.....................Year

M T W T F S Sun
☐ ☐ ☐ ☐ ☐ ☐ ☐

BREAKFAST

Food Item	Serving Size	Carbs	Fats	Protein	Calories

LUNCH

Food Item	Serving Size	Carbs	Fats	Protein	Calories

DINNER

Food Item	Serving Size	Carbs	Fats	Protein	Calories

SNACK

Food Item	Serving Size	Carbs	Fats	Protein	Protein

		Carbs	Fats	Protein	Calories
Total For The Day					

Glasses of Water:

☐ ☐ ☐ ☐ ☐ ☐ ☐ ☐ ☐ ☐ ☐ ☐ ☐

Supplement Intake:	Yes: ☐	No: ☐
Electrolyte Intake:	Yes: ☐	No: ☐
In Ketosis:	Yes: ☐	No: ☐
Exercise:	Yes: ☐	No: ☐

Comments

.... Day.....................Month......................Year

M T W T F S Sun
☐ ☐ ☐ ☐ ☐ ☐ ☐

BREAKFAST

Food Item	Serving Size	Carbs	Fats	Protein	Calories

LUNCH

Food Item	Serving Size	Carbs	Fats	Protein	Calories

DINNER

Food Item	Serving Size	Carbs	Fats	Protein	Calories

SNACK

Food Item	Serving Size	Carbs	Fats	Protein	Protein

		Carbs	Fats	Protein	Calories
Total For The Day					

Glasses of Water:

☐ ☐ ☐ ☐ ☐ ☐ ☐ ☐ ☐ ☐ ☐ ☐ ☐

Comments

Supplement Intake:	Yes: ☐	No: ☐
Electrolyte Intake:	Yes: ☐	No: ☐
In Ketosis:	Yes: ☐	No: ☐
Exercise:	Yes: ☐	No: ☐

.... Day......................Month......................Year

M T W T F S Sun
☐ ☐ ☐ ☐ ☐ ☐ ☐

BREAKFAST

Food Item	Serving Size	Carbs	Fats	Protein	Calories

LUNCH

Food Item	Serving Size	Carbs	Fats	Protein	Calories

DINNER

Food Item	Serving Size	Carbs	Fats	Protein	Calories

SNACK

Food Item	Serving Size	Carbs	Fats	Protein	Protein

		Carbs	Fats	Protein	Calories
Total For The Day					

Glasses of Water:

☐ ☐ ☐ ☐ ☐ ☐ ☐ ☐ ☐ ☐ ☐ ☐ ☐

Comments

Supplement Intake: Yes: ☐   No: ☐

Electrolyte Intake: Yes: ☐   No: ☐

In Ketosis: Yes: ☐   No: ☐

Exercise: Yes: ☐   No: ☐

.... Day......................Month......................Year

M T W T F S Sun
☐ ☐ ☐ ☐ ☐ ☐ ☐

BREAKFAST

Food Item	Serving Size	Carbs	Fats	Protein	Calories

LUNCH

Food Item	Serving Size	Carbs	Fats	Protein	Calories

DINNER

Food Item	Serving Size	Carbs	Fats	Protein	Calories

SNACK

Food Item	Serving Size	Carbs	Fats	Protein	Protein

Total For The Day		Carbs	Fats	Protein	Calories

Glasses of Water:	Comments
☐ ☐ ☐ ☐ ☐ ☐ ☐ ☐ ☐ ☐ ☐ ☐ ☐	

Supplement Intake:	Yes: ☐	No: ☐	
Electrolyte Intake:	Yes: ☐	No: ☐	
In Ketosis:	Yes: ☐	No: ☐	
Exercise:	Yes: ☐	No: ☐	

.... Day.....................Month......................Year

M T W T F S Sun
☐ ☐ ☐ ☐ ☐ ☐ ☐

BREAKFAST

Food Item	Serving Size	Carbs	Fats	Protein	Calories

LUNCH

Food Item	Serving Size	Carbs	Fats	Protein	Calories

DINNER

Food Item	Serving Size	Carbs	Fats	Protein	Calories

SNACK

Food Item	Serving Size	Carbs	Fats	Protein	Protein

		Carbs	Fats	Protein	Calories
Total For The Day					

Glasses of Water:

☐ ☐ ☐ ☐ ☐ ☐ ☐ ☐ ☐ ☐ ☐ ☐ ☐

				Comments
Supplement Intake:	Yes: ☐	No: ☐		
Electrolyte Intake:	Yes: ☐	No: ☐		
In Ketosis:	Yes: ☐	No: ☐		
Exercise:	Yes: ☐	No: ☐		

.... Day....................Month......................Year

M T W T F S Sun
☐ ☐ ☐ ☐ ☐ ☐ ☐

BREAKFAST

Food Item	Serving Size	Carbs	Fats	Protein	Calories

LUNCH

Food Item	Serving Size	Carbs	Fats	Protein	Calories

DINNER

Food Item	Serving Size	Carbs	Fats	Protein	Calories

SNACK

Food Item	Serving Size	Carbs	Fats	Protein	Protein

		Carbs	Fats	Protein	Calories
Total For The Day					

Glasses of Water:	Comments
☐ ☐ ☐ ☐ ☐ ☐ ☐ ☐ ☐ ☐ ☐ ☐	

Supplement Intake:	Yes: ☐	No: ☐	
Electrolyte Intake:	Yes: ☐	No: ☐	
In Ketosis:	Yes: ☐	No: ☐	
Exercise:	Yes: ☐	No: ☐	

.... Day.....................Month.....................Year

M T W T F S Sun
☐ ☐ ☐ ☐ ☐ ☐ ☐

BREAKFAST

Food Item	Serving Size	Carbs	Fats	Protein	Calories

LUNCH

Food Item	Serving Size	Carbs	Fats	Protein	Calories

DINNER

Food Item	Serving Size	Carbs	Fats	Protein	Calories

SNACK

Food Item	Serving Size	Carbs	Fats	Protein	Protein

		Carbs	Fats	Protein	Calories
Total For The Day					

Glasses of Water:
☐ ☐ ☐ ☐ ☐ ☐ ☐ ☐ ☐ ☐ ☐ ☐ ☐

Supplement Intake:	Yes: ☐	No: ☐
Electrolyte Intake:	Yes: ☐	No: ☐
In Ketosis:	Yes: ☐	No: ☐
Exercise:	Yes: ☐	No: ☐

Comments

.... Day......................Month......................Year

M T W T F S Sun
☐ ☐ ☐ ☐ ☐ ☐ ☐

BREAKFAST

Food Item	Serving Size	Carbs	Fats	Protein	Calories

LUNCH

Food Item	Serving Size	Carbs	Fats	Protein	Calories

DINNER

Food Item	Serving Size	Carbs	Fats	Protein	Calories

SNACK

Food Item	Serving Size	Carbs	Fats	Protein	Protein

		Carbs	Fats	Protein	Calories
Total For The Day					

Glasses of Water:	Comments
☐ ☐ ☐ ☐ ☐ ☐ ☐ ☐ ☐ ☐ ☐ ☐ ☐	

Supplement Intake: Yes: ☐ No: ☐

Electrolyte Intake: Yes: ☐ No: ☐

In Ketosis: Yes: ☐ No: ☐

Exercise: Yes: ☐ No: ☐

.... Day.....................Month.....................Year

M T W T F S Sun
☐ ☐ ☐ ☐ ☐ ☐ ☐

BREAKFAST

Food Item	Serving Size	Carbs	Fats	Protein	Calories

LUNCH

Food Item	Serving Size	Carbs	Fats	Protein	Calories

DINNER

Food Item	Serving Size	Carbs	Fats	Protein	Calories

SNACK

Food Item	Serving Size	Carbs	Fats	Protein	Protein

		Carbs	Fats	Protein	Calories
Total For The Day					

Glasses of Water:

☐ ☐ ☐ ☐ ☐ ☐ ☐ ☐ ☐ ☐ ☐ ☐ ☐

Supplement Intake:	Yes: ☐	No: ☐
Electrolyte Intake:	Yes: ☐	No: ☐
In Ketosis:	Yes: ☐	No: ☐
Exercise:	Yes: ☐	No: ☐

Comments

.... Day......................Month......................Year

M T W T F S Sun
☐ ☐ ☐ ☐ ☐ ☐ ☐

BREAKFAST

Food Item	Serving Size	Carbs	Fats	Protein	Calories

LUNCH

Food Item	Serving Size	Carbs	Fats	Protein	Calories

DINNER

Food Item	Serving Size	Carbs	Fats	Protein	Calories

SNACK

Food Item	Serving Size	Carbs	Fats	Protein	Protein

		Carbs	Fats	Protein	Calories
Total For The Day					

Glasses of Water:

☐ ☐ ☐ ☐ ☐ ☐ ☐ ☐ ☐ ☐ ☐ ☐ ☐

Comments

Supplement Intake:	Yes: ☐	No: ☐
Electrolyte Intake:	Yes: ☐	No: ☐
In Ketosis:	Yes: ☐	No: ☐
Exercise:	Yes: ☐	No: ☐

.... Day.......................Month.......................Year

M T W T F S Sun
☐ ☐ ☐ ☐ ☐ ☐ ☐

BREAKFAST

Food Item	Serving Size	Carbs	Fats	Protein	Calories

LUNCH

Food Item	Serving Size	Carbs	Fats	Protein	Calories

DINNER

Food Item	Serving Size	Carbs	Fats	Protein	Calories

SNACK

Food Item	Serving Size	Carbs	Fats	Protein	Protein

Total For The Day		Carbs	Fats	Protein	Calories

Glasses of Water:

☐ ☐ ☐ ☐ ☐ ☐ ☐ ☐ ☐ ☐ ☐ ☐ ☐

				Comments
Supplement Intake:	Yes: ☐	No: ☐		
Electrolyte Intake:	Yes: ☐	No: ☐		
In Ketosis:	Yes: ☐	No: ☐		
Exercise:	Yes: ☐	No: ☐		

.... Day.......................Month.......................Year

M T W T F S Sun
☐ ☐ ☐ ☐ ☐ ☐ ☐

BREAKFAST

Food Item	Serving Size	Carbs	Fats	Protein	Calories

LUNCH

Food Item	Serving Size	Carbs	Fats	Protein	Calories

DINNER

Food Item	Serving Size	Carbs	Fats	Protein	Calories

SNACK

Food Item	Serving Size	Carbs	Fats	Protein	Protein

		Carbs	Fats	Protein	Calories
Total For The Day					

Glasses of Water:	Comments
☐ ☐ ☐ ☐ ☐ ☐ ☐ ☐ ☐ ☐ ☐ ☐ ☐	

Supplement Intake:	Yes: ☐	No: ☐
Electrolyte Intake:	Yes: ☐	No: ☐
In Ketosis:	Yes: ☐	No: ☐
Exercise:	Yes: ☐	No: ☐

.... Day...................Month.....................Year

M T W T F S Sun
☐ ☐ ☐ ☐ ☐ ☐ ☐

BREAKFAST

Food Item	Serving Size	Carbs	Fats	Protein	Calories

LUNCH

Food Item	Serving Size	Carbs	Fats	Protein	Calories

DINNER

Food Item	Serving Size	Carbs	Fats	Protein	Calories

SNACK

Food Item	Serving Size	Carbs	Fats	Protein	Protein

		Carbs	Fats	Protein	Calories
Total For The Day					

Glasses of Water:

☐ ☐ ☐ ☐ ☐ ☐ ☐ ☐ ☐ ☐ ☐ ☐ ☐

Comments

Supplement Intake:	Yes: ☐	No: ☐
Electrolyte Intake:	Yes: ☐	No: ☐
In Ketosis:	Yes: ☐	No: ☐
Exercise:	Yes: ☐	No: ☐

.... Day.....................Month......................Year

M T W T F S Sun
☐ ☐ ☐ ☐ ☐ ☐ ☐

BREAKFAST

Food Item	Serving Size	Carbs	Fats	Protein	Calories

LUNCH

Food Item	Serving Size	Carbs	Fats	Protein	Calories

DINNER

Food Item	Serving Size	Carbs	Fats	Protein	Calories

SNACK

Food Item	Serving Size	Carbs	Fats	Protein	Protein

		Carbs	Fats	Protein	Calories
Total For The Day					

Glasses of Water:

☐ ☐ ☐ ☐ ☐ ☐ ☐ ☐ ☐ ☐ ☐ ☐ ☐

Comments

Supplement Intake:	Yes: ☐	No: ☐
Electrolyte Intake:	Yes: ☐	No: ☐
In Ketosis:	Yes: ☐	No: ☐
Exercise:	Yes: ☐	No: ☐

.... Day.....................Month.....................Year

M T W T F S Sun
☐ ☐ ☐ ☐ ☐ ☐ ☐

BREAKFAST

Food Item	Serving Size	Carbs	Fats	Protein	Calories

LUNCH

Food Item	Serving Size	Carbs	Fats	Protein	Calories

DINNER

Food Item	Serving Size	Carbs	Fats	Protein	Calories

SNACK

Food Item	Serving Size	Carbs	Fats	Protein	Protein

Total For The Day		Carbs	Fats	Protein	Calories

Glasses of Water:	Comments
☐ ☐ ☐ ☐ ☐ ☐ ☐ ☐ ☐ ☐ ☐ ☐ ☐	
Supplement Intake: Yes: ☐ No: ☐	
Electrolyte Intake: Yes: ☐ No: ☐	
In Ketosis: Yes: ☐ No: ☐	
Exercise: Yes: ☐ No: ☐	

.... Day......................Month......................Year

M T W T F S Sun
☐ ☐ ☐ ☐ ☐ ☐ ☐

BREAKFAST

Food Item	Serving Size	Carbs	Fats	Protein	Calories

LUNCH

Food Item	Serving Size	Carbs	Fats	Protein	Calories

DINNER

Food Item	Serving Size	Carbs	Fats	Protein	Calories

SNACK

Food Item	Serving Size	Carbs	Fats	Protein	Protein

		Carbs	Fats	Protein	Calories
Total For The Day					

Glasses of Water:

☐ ☐ ☐ ☐ ☐ ☐ ☐ ☐ ☐ ☐ ☐ ☐ ☐

Comments

Supplement Intake:	Yes: ☐	No: ☐	
Electrolyte Intake:	Yes: ☐	No: ☐	
In Ketosis:	Yes: ☐	No: ☐	
Exercise:	Yes: ☐	No: ☐	

.... Day.....................Month......................Year

M T W T F S Sun
☐ ☐ ☐ ☐ ☐ ☐ ☐

BREAKFAST

Food Item	Serving Size	Carbs	Fats	Protein	Calories

LUNCH

Food Item	Serving Size	Carbs	Fats	Protein	Calories

DINNER

Food Item	Serving Size	Carbs	Fats	Protein	Calories

SNACK

Food Item	Serving Size	Carbs	Fats	Protein	Protein

		Carbs	Fats	Protein	Calories
Total For The Day					

Glasses of Water:

☐ ☐ ☐ ☐ ☐ ☐ ☐ ☐ ☐ ☐ ☐ ☐ ☐

Comments

Supplement Intake:	Yes: ☐	No: ☐	
Electrolyte Intake:	Yes: ☐	No: ☐	
In Ketosis:	Yes: ☐	No: ☐	
Exercise:	Yes: ☐	No: ☐	

.... Day.....................Month......................Year

M T W T F S Sun
☐ ☐ ☐ ☐ ☐ ☐ ☐

BREAKFAST

Food Item	Serving Size	Carbs	Fats	Protein	Calories

LUNCH

Food Item	Serving Size	Carbs	Fats	Protein	Calories

DINNER

Food Item	Serving Size	Carbs	Fats	Protein	Calories

SNACK

Food Item	Serving Size	Carbs	Fats	Protein	Protein

Total For The Day		Carbs	Fats	Protein	Calories

Glasses of Water:	Comments
☐ ☐ ☐ ☐ ☐ ☐ ☐ ☐ ☐ ☐ ☐ ☐ ☐	

Supplement Intake:	Yes: ☐	No: ☐	
Electrolyte Intake:	Yes: ☐	No: ☐	
In Ketosis:	Yes: ☐	No: ☐	
Exercise:	Yes: ☐	No: ☐	

.... Day.....................Month.....................Year

M T W T F S Sun

☐ ☐ ☐ ☐ ☐ ☐ ☐

BREAKFAST

Food Item	Serving Size	Carbs	Fats	Protein	Calories

LUNCH

Food Item	Serving Size	Carbs	Fats	Protein	Calories

DINNER

Food Item	Serving Size	Carbs	Fats	Protein	Calories

SNACK

Food Item	Serving Size	Carbs	Fats	Protein	Protein

		Carbs	Fats	Protein	Calories
Total For The Day					

Glasses of Water:	Comments
☐ ☐ ☐ ☐ ☐ ☐ ☐ ☐ ☐ ☐ ☐ ☐ ☐	

Supplement Intake:	Yes: ☐	No: ☐
Electrolyte Intake:	Yes: ☐	No: ☐
In Ketosis:	Yes: ☐	No: ☐
Exercise:	Yes: ☐	No: ☐

.... Day......................Month......................Year

M T W T F S Sun
☐ ☐ ☐ ☐ ☐ ☐ ☐

BREAKFAST

Food Item	Serving Size	Carbs	Fats	Protein	Calories

LUNCH

Food Item	Serving Size	Carbs	Fats	Protein	Calories

DINNER

Food Item	Serving Size	Carbs	Fats	Protein	Calories

SNACK

Food Item	Serving Size	Carbs	Fats	Protein	Protein

		Carbs	Fats	Protein	Calories
Total For The Day					

Glasses of Water:	Comments
☐ ☐ ☐ ☐ ☐ ☐ ☐ ☐ ☐ ☐ ☐ ☐ ☐	
Supplement Intake: Yes: ☐ No: ☐	
Electrolyte Intake: Yes: ☐ No: ☐	
In Ketosis: Yes: ☐ No: ☐	
Exercise: Yes: ☐ No: ☐	

.... Day......................Month......................Year

M T W T F S Sun
☐ ☐ ☐ ☐ ☐ ☐ ☐

BREAKFAST

Food Item	Serving Size	Carbs	Fats	Protein	Calories

LUNCH

Food Item	Serving Size	Carbs	Fats	Protein	Calories

DINNER

Food Item	Serving Size	Carbs	Fats	Protein	Calories

SNACK

Food Item	Serving Size	Carbs	Fats	Protein	Protein

		Carbs	Fats	Protein	Calories
Total For The Day					

Glasses of Water:

☐ ☐ ☐ ☐ ☐ ☐ ☐ ☐ ☐ ☐ ☐ ☐ ☐

Comments

Supplement Intake:	Yes: ☐	No: ☐
Electrolyte Intake:	Yes: ☐	No: ☐
In Ketosis:	Yes: ☐	No: ☐
Exercise:	Yes: ☐	No: ☐

.... Day.....................Month......................Year

M T W T F S Sun
☐ ☐ ☐ ☐ ☐ ☐ ☐

BREAKFAST

Food Item	Serving Size	Carbs	Fats	Protein	Calories

LUNCH

Food Item	Serving Size	Carbs	Fats	Protein	Calories

DINNER

Food Item	Serving Size	Carbs	Fats	Protein	Calories

SNACK

Food Item	Serving Size	Carbs	Fats	Protein	Protein

		Carbs	Fats	Protein	Calories
Total For The Day					

Glasses of Water:

☐ ☐ ☐ ☐ ☐ ☐ ☐ ☐ ☐ ☐ ☐ ☐ ☐ ☐

Comments

Supplement Intake:	Yes: ☐	No: ☐
Electrolyte Intake:	Yes: ☐	No: ☐
In Ketosis:	Yes: ☐	No: ☐
Exercise:	Yes: ☐	No: ☐

.... Day......................Month.....................Year

M T W T F S Sun
☐ ☐ ☐ ☐ ☐ ☐ ☐

BREAKFAST

Food Item	Serving Size	Carbs	Fats	Protein	Calories

LUNCH

Food Item	Serving Size	Carbs	Fats	Protein	Calories

DINNER

Food Item	Serving Size	Carbs	Fats	Protein	Calories

SNACK

Food Item	Serving Size	Carbs	Fats	Protein	Protein

		Carbs	Fats	Protein	Calories
Total For The Day					

Glasses of Water:
☐ ☐ ☐ ☐ ☐ ☐ ☐ ☐ ☐ ☐ ☐ ☐

Supplement Intake:	Yes: ☐	No: ☐
Electrolyte Intake:	Yes: ☐	No: ☐
In Ketosis:	Yes: ☐	No: ☐
Exercise:	Yes: ☐	No: ☐

Comments

.... Day.....................Month.....................Year

M T W T F S Sun
☐ ☐ ☐ ☐ ☐ ☐ ☐

BREAKFAST

Food Item	Serving Size	Carbs	Fats	Protein	Calories

LUNCH

Food Item	Serving Size	Carbs	Fats	Protein	Calories

DINNER

Food Item	Serving Size	Carbs	Fats	Protein	Calories

SNACK

Food Item	Serving Size	Carbs	Fats	Protein	Protein

		Carbs	Fats	Protein	Calories
Total For The Day					

Glasses of Water:	Comments
☐ ☐ ☐ ☐ ☐ ☐ ☐ ☐ ☐ ☐ ☐ ☐ ☐	
Supplement Intake: Yes: ☐ No: ☐	
Electrolyte Intake: Yes: ☐ No: ☐	
In Ketosis: Yes: ☐ No: ☐	
Exercise: Yes: ☐ No: ☐	

.... Day.....................Month.....................Year

M T W T F S Sun
☐ ☐ ☐ ☐ ☐ ☐ ☐

BREAKFAST

Food Item	Serving Size	Carbs	Fats	Protein	Calories

LUNCH

Food Item	Serving Size	Carbs	Fats	Protein	Calories
				.	

DINNER

Food Item	Serving Size	Carbs	Fats	Protein	Calories

SNACK

Food Item	Serving Size	Carbs	Fats	Protein	Protein

		Carbs	Fats	Protein	Calories
Total For The Day					

Glasses of Water:

☐ ☐ ☐ ☐ ☐ ☐ ☐ ☐ ☐ ☐ ☐ ☐ ☐

Comments

Supplement Intake:	Yes: ☐	No: ☐
Electrolyte Intake:	Yes: ☐	No: ☐
In Ketosis:	Yes: ☐	No: ☐
Exercise:	Yes: ☐	No: ☐

.... Day.....................Month.......................Year

M T W T F S Sun
☐ ☐ ☐ ☐ ☐ ☐ ☐

BREAKFAST

Food Item	Serving Size	Carbs	Fats	Protein	Calories

LUNCH

Food Item	Serving Size	Carbs	Fats	Protein	Calories

DINNER

Food Item	Serving Size	Carbs	Fats	Protein	Calories

SNACK

Food Item	Serving Size	Carbs	Fats	Protein	Protein

		Carbs	Fats	Protein	Calories
Total For The Day					

Glasses of Water:	Comments
☐ ☐ ☐ ☐ ☐ ☐ ☐ ☐ ☐ ☐ ☐ ☐ ☐ ☐	

Supplement Intake:	Yes: ☐	No: ☐
Electrolyte Intake:	Yes: ☐	No: ☐
In Ketosis:	Yes: ☐	No: ☐
Exercise:	Yes: ☐	No: ☐

.... Day.....................Month.....................Year

M T W T F S Sun
☐ ☐ ☐ ☐ ☐ ☐ ☐

BREAKFAST

Food Item	Serving Size	Carbs	Fats	Protein	Calories

LUNCH

Food Item	Serving Size	Carbs	Fats	Protein	Calories

DINNER

Food Item	Serving Size	Carbs	Fats	Protein	Calories

SNACK

Food Item	Serving Size	Carbs	Fats	Protein	Protein

		Carbs	Fats	Protein	Calories
Total For The Day					

Glasses of Water:

☐ ☐ ☐ ☐ ☐ ☐ ☐ ☐ ☐ ☐ ☐ ☐ ☐

			Comments
Supplement Intake:	Yes: ☐	No: ☐	
Electrolyte Intake:	Yes: ☐	No: ☐	
In Ketosis:	Yes: ☐	No: ☐	
Exercise:	Yes: ☐	No: ☐	

.... Day..................... Month..................... Year

M T W T F S Sun
☐ ☐ ☐ ☐ ☐ ☐ ☐

BREAKFAST

Food Item	Serving Size	Carbs	Fats	Protein	Calories

LUNCH

Food Item	Serving Size	Carbs	Fats	Protein	Calories

DINNER

Food Item	Serving Size	Carbs	Fats	Protein	Calories

SNACK

Food Item	Serving Size	Carbs	Fats	Protein	Protein

Total For The Day		Carbs	Fats	Protein	Calories

Glasses of Water:	Comments
☐ ☐ ☐ ☐ ☐ ☐ ☐ ☐ ☐ ☐ ☐ ☐ ☐	
Supplement Intake: Yes: ☐ No: ☐	
Electrolyte Intake: Yes: ☐ No: ☐	
In Ketosis: Yes: ☐ No: ☐	
Exercise: Yes: ☐ No: ☐	

M T W T F S Sun
☐ ☐ ☐ ☐ ☐ ☐ ☐

.... Day......................Month......................Year

BREAKFAST

Food Item	Serving Size	Carbs	Fats	Protein	Calories

LUNCH

Food Item	Serving Size	Carbs	Fats	Protein	Calories

DINNER

Food Item	Serving Size	Carbs	Fats	Protein	Calories

SNACK

Food Item	Serving Size	Carbs	Fats	Protein	Protein

		Carbs	Fats	Protein	Calories
Total For The Day					

Glasses of Water:	Comments
☐ ☐ ☐ ☐ ☐ ☐ ☐ ☐ ☐ ☐ ☐ ☐ ☐	
Supplement Intake: Yes: ☐ No: ☐	
Electrolyte Intake: Yes: ☐ No: ☐	
In Ketosis: Yes: ☐ No: ☐	
Exercise: Yes: ☐ No: ☐	

.... Day.....................Month.....................Year

M T W T F S Sun
☐ ☐ ☐ ☐ ☐ ☐ ☐

BREAKFAST

Food Item	Serving Size	Carbs	Fats	Protein	Calories

LUNCH

Food Item	Serving Size	Carbs	Fats	Protein	Calories

DINNER

Food Item	Serving Size	Carbs	Fats	Protein	Calories

SNACK

Food Item	Serving Size	Carbs	Fats	Protein	Protein

Total For The Day		Carbs	Fats	Protein	Calories

Glasses of Water:

☐ ☐ ☐ ☐ ☐ ☐ ☐ ☐ ☐ ☐ ☐ ☐ ☐

Supplement Intake:	Yes: ☐	No: ☐
Electrolyte Intake:	Yes: ☐	No: ☐
In Ketosis:	Yes: ☐	No: ☐
Exercise:	Yes: ☐	No: ☐

Comments

.... Day.................Month.................Year

M T W T F S Sun
☐ ☐ ☐ ☐ ☐ ☐ ☐

BREAKFAST

Food Item	Serving Size	Carbs	Fats	Protein	Calories

LUNCH

Food Item	Serving Size	Carbs	Fats	Protein	Calories

DINNER

Food Item	Serving Size	Carbs	Fats	Protein	Calories

SNACK

Food Item	Serving Size	Carbs	Fats	Protein	Protein

Total For The Day		Carbs	Fats	Protein	Calories

Glasses of Water:

☐ ☐ ☐ ☐ ☐ ☐ ☐ ☐ ☐ ☐ ☐ ☐ ☐

Supplement Intake:	Yes: ☐	No: ☐
Electrolyte Intake:	Yes: ☐	No: ☐
In Ketosis:	Yes: ☐	No: ☐
Exercise:	Yes: ☐	No: ☐

Comments

.... Day.....................Month......................Year

M T W T F S Sun
☐ ☐ ☐ ☐ ☐ ☐ ☐

BREAKFAST

Food Item	Serving Size	Carbs	Fats	Protein	Calories

LUNCH

Food Item	Serving Size	Carbs	Fats	Protein	Calories

DINNER

Food Item	Serving Size	Carbs	Fats	Protein	Calories

SNACK

Food Item	Serving Size	Carbs	Fats	Protein	Protein

		Carbs	Fats	Protein	Calories
Total For The Day					

Glasses of Water:	Comments
☐ ☐ ☐ ☐ ☐ ☐ ☐ ☐ ☐ ☐ ☐ ☐ ☐	

Supplement Intake:	Yes: ☐	No: ☐	
Electrolyte Intake:	Yes: ☐	No: ☐	
In Ketosis:	Yes: ☐	No: ☐	
Exercise:	Yes: ☐	No: ☐	

.... Day.......................Month.......................Year

M T W T F S Sun
☐ ☐ ☐ ☐ ☐ ☐ ☐

BREAKFAST

Food Item	Serving Size	Carbs	Fats	Protein	Calories

LUNCH

Food Item	Serving Size	Carbs	Fats	Protein	Calories

DINNER

Food Item	Serving Size	Carbs	Fats	Protein	Calories

SNACK

Food Item	Serving Size	Carbs	Fats	Protein	Protein

		Carbs	Fats	Protein	Calories
Total For The Day					

Glasses of Water:

☐ ☐ ☐ ☐ ☐ ☐ ☐ ☐ ☐ ☐ ☐ ☐ ☐ ☐

Comments

Supplement Intake:	Yes: ☐	No: ☐
Electrolyte Intake:	Yes: ☐	No: ☐
In Ketosis:	Yes: ☐	No: ☐
Exercise:	Yes: ☐	No: ☐

.... Day.....................Month.....................Year

M T W T F S Sun
☐ ☐ ☐ ☐ ☐ ☐ ☐

BREAKFAST

Food Item	Serving Size	Carbs	Fats	Protein	Calories

LUNCH

Food Item	Serving Size	Carbs	Fats	Protein	Calories

DINNER

Food Item	Serving Size	Carbs	Fats	Protein	Calories

SNACK

Food Item	Serving Size	Carbs	Fats	Protein	Protein

Total For The Day		Carbs	Fats	Protein	Calories

Glasses of Water:

☐ ☐ ☐ ☐ ☐ ☐ ☐ ☐ ☐ ☐ ☐ ☐ ☐

| **Comments** |

Supplement Intake: Yes: ☐   No: ☐

Electrolyte Intake: Yes: ☐   No: ☐

In Ketosis: Yes: ☐   No: ☐

Exercise: Yes: ☐   No: ☐

.... Day.....................Month......................Year

M T W T F S Sun
☐ ☐ ☐ ☐ ☐ ☐ ☐

BREAKFAST

Food Item	Serving Size	Carbs	Fats	Protein	Calories

LUNCH

Food Item	Serving Size	Carbs	Fats	Protein	Calories

DINNER

Food Item	Serving Size	Carbs	Fats	Protein	Calories

SNACK

Food Item	Serving Size	Carbs	Fats	Protein	Protein

		Carbs	Fats	Protein	Calories
Total For The Day					

Glasses of Water:
☐ ☐ ☐ ☐ ☐ ☐ ☐ ☐ ☐ ☐ ☐ ☐ ☐

Comments

Supplement Intake:	Yes: ☐	No: ☐
Electrolyte Intake:	Yes: ☐	No: ☐
In Ketosis:	Yes: ☐	No: ☐
Exercise:	Yes: ☐	No: ☐

.... Day.....................Month.......................Year

M T W T F S Sun
☐ ☐ ☐ ☐ ☐ ☐ ☐

BREAKFAST

Food Item	Serving Size	Carbs	Fats	Protein	Calories

LUNCH

Food Item	Serving Size	Carbs	Fats	Protein	Calories

DINNER

Food Item	Serving Size	Carbs	Fats	Protein	Calories

SNACK

Food Item	Serving Size	Carbs	Fats	Protein	Protein

		Carbs	Fats	Protein	Calories
Total For The Day					

Glasses of Water:	Comments
☐ ☐ ☐ ☐ ☐ ☐ ☐ ☐ ☐ ☐ ☐ ☐ ☐	
Supplement Intake: Yes: ☐ No: ☐	
Electrolyte Intake: Yes: ☐ No: ☐	
In Ketosis: Yes: ☐ No: ☐	
Exercise: Yes: ☐ No: ☐	

.... Day.....................Month.....................Year

M T W T F S Sun
☐ ☐ ☐ ☐ ☐ ☐ ☐

BREAKFAST

Food Item	Serving Size	Carbs	Fats	Protein	Calories

LUNCH

Food Item	Serving Size	Carbs	Fats	Protein	Calories

DINNER

Food Item	Serving Size	Carbs	Fats	Protein	Calories

SNACK

Food Item	Serving Size	Carbs	Fats	Protein	Protein

		Carbs	Fats	Protein	Calories
Total For The Day					

Glasses of Water:

☐ ☐ ☐ ☐ ☐ ☐ ☐ ☐ ☐ ☐ ☐ ☐ ☐

Comments

Supplement Intake:	Yes: ☐	No: ☐
Electrolyte Intake:	Yes: ☐	No: ☐
In Ketosis:	Yes: ☐	No: ☐
Exercise:	Yes: ☐	No: ☐

.... Day..................... Month..................... Year

M T W T F S Sun
☐ ☐ ☐ ☐ ☐ ☐ ☐

BREAKFAST

Food Item	Serving Size	Carbs	Fats	Protein	Calories

LUNCH

Food Item	Serving Size	Carbs	Fats	Protein	Calories

DINNER

Food Item	Serving Size	Carbs	Fats	Protein	Calories

SNACK

Food Item	Serving Size	Carbs	Fats	Protein	Protein

		Carbs	Fats	Protein	Calories
Total For The Day					

Glasses of Water:	Comments
☐ ☐ ☐ ☐ ☐ ☐ ☐ ☐ ☐ ☐ ☐ ☐ ☐	
Supplement Intake: Yes: ☐ No: ☐	
Electrolyte Intake: Yes: ☐ No: ☐	
In Ketosis: Yes: ☐ No: ☐	
Exercise: Yes: ☐ No: ☐	

.... Day......................Month......................Year

M T W T F S Sun
☐ ☐ ☐ ☐ ☐ ☐ ☐

BREAKFAST

Food Item	Serving Size	Carbs	Fats	Protein	Calories

LUNCH

Food Item	Serving Size	Carbs	Fats	Protein	Calories

DINNER

Food Item	Serving Size	Carbs	Fats	Protein	Calories

SNACK

Food Item	Serving Size	Carbs	Fats	Protein	Protein

		Carbs	Fats	Protein	Calories
Total For The Day					

Glasses of Water:	Comments
☐ ☐ ☐ ☐ ☐ ☐ ☐ ☐ ☐ ☐ ☐ ☐ ☐	

Supplement Intake:	Yes: ☐	No: ☐	
Electrolyte Intake:	Yes: ☐	No: ☐	
In Ketosis:	Yes: ☐	No: ☐	
Exercise:	Yes: ☐	No: ☐	

.... Day.....................Month.....................Year

M T W T F S Sun
☐ ☐ ☐ ☐ ☐ ☐ ☐

BREAKFAST

Food Item	Serving Size	Carbs	Fats	Protein	Calories

LUNCH

Food Item	Serving Size	Carbs	Fats	Protein	Calories

DINNER

Food Item	Serving Size	Carbs	Fats	Protein	Calories

SNACK

Food Item	Serving Size	Carbs	Fats	Protein	Protein

		Carbs	Fats	Protein	Calories
Total For The Day					

Glasses of Water:	Comments
☐ ☐ ☐ ☐ ☐ ☐ ☐ ☐ ☐ ☐ ☐ ☐ ☐	

Supplement Intake:	Yes: ☐	No: ☐	
Electrolyte Intake:	Yes: ☐	No: ☐	
In Ketosis:	Yes: ☐	No: ☐	
Exercise:	Yes: ☐	No: ☐	

.... Day......................Month......................Year

M T W T F S Sun
☐ ☐ ☐ ☐ ☐ ☐ ☐

BREAKFAST

Food Item	Serving Size	Carbs	Fats	Protein	Calories

LUNCH

Food Item	Serving Size	Carbs	Fats	Protein	Calories

DINNER

Food Item	Serving Size	Carbs	Fats	Protein	Calories

SNACK

Food Item	Serving Size	Carbs	Fats	Protein	Protein

		Carbs	Fats	Protein	Calories
Total For The Day					

Glasses of Water:

☐ ☐ ☐ ☐ ☐ ☐ ☐ ☐ ☐ ☐ ☐ ☐ ☐

Comments

Supplement Intake:	Yes: ☐	No: ☐
Electrolyte Intake:	Yes: ☐	No: ☐
In Ketosis:	Yes: ☐	No: ☐
Exercise:	Yes: ☐	No: ☐

.... Day.....................Month.......................Year

M T W T F S Sun
☐ ☐ ☐ ☐ ☐ ☐ ☐

BREAKFAST

Food Item	Serving Size	Carbs	Fats	Protein	Calories

LUNCH

Food Item	Serving Size	Carbs	Fats	Protein	Calories

DINNER

Food Item	Serving Size	Carbs	Fats	Protein	Calories

SNACK

Food Item	Serving Size	Carbs	Fats	Protein	Protein

		Carbs	Fats	Protein	Calories
Total For The Day					

Glasses of Water:

☐ ☐ ☐ ☐ ☐ ☐ ☐ ☐ ☐ ☐ ☐ ☐ ☐ ☐

Supplement Intake:	Yes: ☐	No: ☐
Electrolyte Intake:	Yes: ☐	No: ☐
In Ketosis:	Yes: ☐	No: ☐
Exercise:	Yes: ☐	No: ☐

Comments

.... Day.....................Month.....................Year

M T W T F S Sun
☐ ☐ ☐ ☐ ☐ ☐ ☐

BREAKFAST

Food Item	Serving Size	Carbs	Fats	Protein	Calories

LUNCH

Food Item	Serving Size	Carbs	Fats	Protein	Calories

DINNER

Food Item	Serving Size	Carbs	Fats	Protein	Calories

SNACK

Food Item	Serving Size	Carbs	Fats	Protein	Protein

		Carbs	Fats	Protein	Calories
Total For The Day					

Glasses of Water:
☐ ☐ ☐ ☐ ☐ ☐ ☐ ☐ ☐ ☐ ☐ ☐ ☐

Supplement Intake:	Yes: ☐	No: ☐	
Electrolyte Intake:	Yes: ☐	No: ☐	
In Ketosis:	Yes: ☐	No: ☐	
Exercise:	Yes: ☐	No: ☐	

Comments

.... Day......................Month.......................Year

M T W T F S Sun
☐ ☐ ☐ ☐ ☐ ☐ ☐

BREAKFAST

Food Item	Serving Size	Carbs	Fats	Protein	Calories

LUNCH

Food Item	Serving Size	Carbs	Fats	Protein	Calories

DINNER

Food Item	Serving Size	Carbs	Fats	Protein	Calories

SNACK

Food Item	Serving Size	Carbs	Fats	Protein	Protein

		Carbs	Fats	Protein	Calories
Total For The Day					

Glasses of Water:
☐ ☐ ☐ ☐ ☐ ☐ ☐ ☐ ☐ ☐ ☐ ☐ ☐

Supplement Intake:	Yes: ☐	No: ☐
Electrolyte Intake:	Yes: ☐	No: ☐
In Ketosis:	Yes: ☐	No: ☐
Exercise:	Yes: ☐	No: ☐

Comments

.... Day......................Month......................Year

M T W T F S Sun
☐ ☐ ☐ ☐ ☐ ☐ ☐

BREAKFAST

Food Item	Serving Size	Carbs	Fats	Protein	Calories

LUNCH

Food Item	Serving Size	Carbs	Fats	Protein	Calories

DINNER

Food Item	Serving Size	Carbs	Fats	Protein	Calories

SNACK

Food Item	Serving Size	Carbs	Fats	Protein	Protein

		Carbs	Fats	Protein	Calories
Total For The Day					

Glasses of Water:	Comments
☐ ☐ ☐ ☐ ☐ ☐ ☐ ☐ ☐ ☐ ☐ ☐ ☐	

Supplement Intake:	Yes: ☐	No: ☐	
Electrolyte Intake:	Yes: ☐	No: ☐	
In Ketosis:	Yes: ☐	No: ☐	
Exercise:	Yes: ☐	No: ☐	

.... Day......................Month......................Year

M T W T F S Sun
☐ ☐ ☐ ☐ ☐ ☐ ☐

BREAKFAST

Food Item	Serving Size	Carbs	Fats	Protein	Calories

LUNCH

Food Item	Serving Size	Carbs	Fats	Protein	Calories

DINNER

Food Item	Serving Size	Carbs	Fats	Protein	Calories

SNACK

Food Item	Serving Size	Carbs	Fats	Protein	Protein

		Carbs	Fats	Protein	Calories
Total For The Day					

Glasses of Water:	Comments
☐ ☐ ☐ ☐ ☐ ☐ ☐ ☐ ☐ ☐ ☐ ☐ ☐	

Supplement Intake:	Yes: ☐	No: ☐	
Electrolyte Intake:	Yes: ☐	No: ☐	
In Ketosis:	Yes: ☐	No: ☐	
Exercise:	Yes: ☐	No: ☐	

.... Day.....................Month.....................Year

M T W T F S Sun
☐ ☐ ☐ ☐ ☐ ☐ ☐

BREAKFAST

Food Item	Serving Size	Carbs	Fats	Protein	Calories

LUNCH

Food Item	Serving Size	Carbs	Fats	Protein	Calories

DINNER

Food Item	Serving Size	Carbs	Fats	Protein	Calories

SNACK

Food Item	Serving Size	Carbs	Fats	Protein	Protein

		Carbs	Fats	Protein	Calories
Total For The Day					

Glasses of Water:	Comments
☐ ☐ ☐ ☐ ☐ ☐ ☐ ☐ ☐ ☐ ☐ ☐	
Supplement Intake: Yes: ☐ No: ☐	
Electrolyte Intake: Yes: ☐ No: ☐	
In Ketosis: Yes: ☐ No: ☐	
Exercise: Yes: ☐ No: ☐	

.... Day......................Month......................Year

M T W T F S Sun
☐ ☐ ☐ ☐ ☐ ☐ ☐

BREAKFAST

Food Item	Serving Size	Carbs	Fats	Protein	Calories

LUNCH

Food Item	Serving Size	Carbs	Fats	Protein	Calories

DINNER

Food Item	Serving Size	Carbs	Fats	Protein	Calories

SNACK

Food Item	Serving Size	Carbs	Fats	Protein	Protein

		Carbs	Fats	Protein	Calories
Total For The Day					

Glasses of Water:

☐ ☐ ☐ ☐ ☐ ☐ ☐ ☐ ☐ ☐ ☐ ☐

Comments

Supplement Intake:	Yes: ☐	No: ☐
Electrolyte Intake:	Yes: ☐	No: ☐
In Ketosis:	Yes: ☐	No: ☐
Exercise:	Yes: ☐	No: ☐

.... Day .... Month .... Year

M T W T F S Sun
☐ ☐ ☐ ☐ ☐ ☐ ☐

BREAKFAST

Food Item	Serving Size	Carbs	Fats	Protein	Calories

LUNCH

Food Item	Serving Size	Carbs	Fats	Protein	Calories

DINNER

Food Item	Serving Size	Carbs	Fats	Protein	Calories

SNACK

Food Item	Serving Size	Carbs	Fats	Protein	Protein

		Carbs	Fats	Protein	Calories
Total For The Day					

Glasses of Water:

☐ ☐ ☐ ☐ ☐ ☐ ☐ ☐ ☐ ☐ ☐ ☐ ☐

Comments

Supplement Intake:	Yes: ☐	No: ☐
Electrolyte Intake:	Yes: ☐	No: ☐
In Ketosis:	Yes: ☐	No: ☐
Exercise:	Yes: ☐	No: ☐

.... Day.....................Month.....................Year

M T W T F S Sun
□ □ □ □ □ □ □

BREAKFAST

Food Item	Serving Size	Carbs	Fats	Protein	Calories

LUNCH

Food Item	Serving Size	Carbs	Fats	Protein	Calories

DINNER

Food Item	Serving Size	Carbs	Fats	Protein	Calories

SNACK

Food Item	Serving Size	Carbs	Fats	Protein	Protein

		Carbs	Fats	Protein	Calories
Total For The Day					

Glasses of Water:	Comments
□ □ □ □ □ □ □ □ □ □ □ □ □	

Supplement Intake:	Yes: □	No: □	
Electrolyte Intake:	Yes: □	No: □	
In Ketosis:	Yes: □	No: □	
Exercise:	Yes: □	No: □	

.... Day..................... Month..................... Year

M T W T F S Sun
☐ ☐ ☐ ☐ ☐ ☐ ☐

BREAKFAST

Food Item	Serving Size	Carbs	Fats	Protein	Calories

LUNCH

Food Item	Serving Size	Carbs	Fats	Protein	Calories

DINNER

Food Item	Serving Size	Carbs	Fats	Protein	Calories

SNACK

Food Item	Serving Size	Carbs	Fats	Protein	Protein

		Carbs	Fats	Protein	Calories
Total For The Day					

Glasses of Water:	Comments
☐ ☐ ☐ ☐ ☐ ☐ ☐ ☐ ☐ ☐ ☐ ☐	

Supplement Intake:	Yes: ☐	No: ☐
Electrolyte Intake:	Yes: ☐	No: ☐
In Ketosis:	Yes: ☐	No: ☐
Exercise:	Yes: ☐	No: ☐

.... Day.....................Month.......................Year

M T W T F S Sun
☐ ☐ ☐ ☐ ☐ ☐ ☐

BREAKFAST

Food Item	Serving Size	Carbs	Fats	Protein	Calories

LUNCH

Food Item	Serving Size	Carbs	Fats	Protein	Calories

DINNER

Food Item	Serving Size	Carbs	Fats	Protein	Calories

SNACK

Food Item	Serving Size	Carbs	Fats	Protein	Protein

		Carbs	Fats	Protein	Calories
Total For The Day					

Glasses of Water:
☐ ☐ ☐ ☐ ☐ ☐ ☐ ☐ ☐ ☐ ☐ ☐ ☐

Comments

Supplement Intake:	Yes: ☐	No: ☐
Electrolyte Intake:	Yes: ☐	No: ☐
In Ketosis:	Yes: ☐	No: ☐
Exercise:	Yes: ☐	No: ☐

.... Day..................... Month..................... Year

M T W T F S Sun
☐ ☐ ☐ ☐ ☐ ☐ ☐

BREAKFAST

Food Item	Serving Size	Carbs	Fats	Protein	Calories

LUNCH

Food Item	Serving Size	Carbs	Fats	Protein	Calories

DINNER

Food Item	Serving Size	Carbs	Fats	Protein	Calories

SNACK

Food Item	Serving Size	Carbs	Fats	Protein	Protein

		Carbs	Fats	Protein	Calories
Total For The Day					

Glasses of Water:	Comments
☐ ☐ ☐ ☐ ☐ ☐ ☐ ☐ ☐ ☐ ☐ ☐ ☐	

Supplement Intake:	Yes: ☐	No: ☐		
Electrolyte Intake:	Yes: ☐	No: ☐		
In Ketosis:	Yes: ☐	No: ☐		
Exercise:	Yes: ☐	No: ☐		

.... Day.................Month.................Year

M T W T F S Sun
☐ ☐ ☐ ☐ ☐ ☐ ☐

BREAKFAST

Food Item	Serving Size	Carbs	Fats	Protein	Calories

LUNCH

Food Item	Serving Size	Carbs	Fats	Protein	Calories

DINNER

Food Item	Serving Size	Carbs	Fats	Protein	Calories

SNACK

Food Item	Serving Size	Carbs	Fats	Protein	Protein

		Carbs	Fats	Protein	Calories
Total For The Day					

Glasses of Water:
☐ ☐ ☐ ☐ ☐ ☐ ☐ ☐ ☐ ☐ ☐ ☐ ☐

Supplement Intake:	Yes: ☐	No: ☐
Electrolyte Intake:	Yes: ☐	No: ☐
In Ketosis:	Yes: ☐	No: ☐
Exercise:	Yes: ☐	No: ☐

Comments

.... Day......................Month......................Year

M T W T F S Sun
☐ ☐ ☐ ☐ ☐ ☐ ☐

BREAKFAST

Food Item	Serving Size	Carbs	Fats	Protein	Calories

LUNCH

Food Item	Serving Size	Carbs	Fats	Protein	Calories

DINNER

Food Item	Serving Size	Carbs	Fats	Protein	Calories

SNACK

Food Item	Serving Size	Carbs	Fats	Protein	Protein

		Carbs	Fats	Protein	Calories
Total For The Day					

Glasses of Water:	Comments
☐ ☐ ☐ ☐ ☐ ☐ ☐ ☐ ☐ ☐ ☐ ☐	
Supplement Intake: Yes: ☐ No: ☐	
Electrolyte Intake: Yes: ☐ No: ☐	
In Ketosis: Yes: ☐ No: ☐	
Exercise: Yes: ☐ No: ☐	

.... Day.....................Month.....................Year

M T W T F S Sun
☐ ☐ ☐ ☐ ☐ ☐ ☐

BREAKFAST

Food Item	Serving Size	Carbs	Fats	Protein	Calories

LUNCH

Food Item	Serving Size	Carbs	Fats	Protein	Calories

DINNER

Food Item	Serving Size	Carbs	Fats	Protein	Calories

SNACK

Food Item	Serving Size	Carbs	Fats	Protein	Protein

		Carbs	Fats	Protein	Calories
Total For The Day					

Glasses of Water:

☐ ☐ ☐ ☐ ☐ ☐ ☐ ☐ ☐ ☐ ☐ ☐ ☐

Comments

Supplement Intake:	Yes: ☐	No: ☐	
Electrolyte Intake:	Yes: ☐	No: ☐	
In Ketosis:	Yes: ☐	No: ☐	
Exercise:	Yes: ☐	No: ☐	

.... Day.....................Month......................Year

M T W T F S Sun
☐ ☐ ☐ ☐ ☐ ☐ ☐

BREAKFAST

Food Item	Serving Size	Carbs	Fats	Protein	Calories

LUNCH

Food Item	Serving Size	Carbs	Fats	Protein	Calories

DINNER

Food Item	Serving Size	Carbs	Fats	Protein	Calories

SNACK

Food Item	Serving Size	Carbs	Fats	Protein	Protein

		Carbs	Fats	Protein	Calories
Total For The Day					

Glasses of Water:

☐ ☐ ☐ ☐ ☐ ☐ ☐ ☐ ☐ ☐ ☐ ☐

					Comments
Supplement Intake:	Yes: ☐	No: ☐			
Electrolyte Intake:	Yes: ☐	No: ☐			
In Ketosis:	Yes: ☐	No: ☐			
Exercise:	Yes: ☐	No: ☐			

.... Day.....................Month.....................Year

M T W T F S Sun
☐ ☐ ☐ ☐ ☐ ☐ ☐

BREAKFAST

Food Item	Serving Size	Carbs	Fats	Protein	Calories

LUNCH

Food Item	Serving Size	Carbs	Fats	Protein	Calories

DINNER

Food Item	Serving Size	Carbs	Fats	Protein	Calories

SNACK

Food Item	Serving Size	Carbs	Fats	Protein	Protein

		Carbs	Fats	Protein	Calories
Total For The Day					

Glasses of Water:
☐ ☐ ☐ ☐ ☐ ☐ ☐ ☐ ☐ ☐ ☐ ☐ ☐

Supplement Intake:	Yes: ☐	No: ☐
Electrolyte Intake:	Yes: ☐	No: ☐
In Ketosis:	Yes: ☐	No: ☐
Exercise:	Yes: ☐	No: ☐

Comments

.... Day.................... Month..................... Year

M T W T F S Sun
☐ ☐ ☐ ☐ ☐ ☐ ☐

BREAKFAST

Food Item	Serving Size	Carbs	Fats	Protein	Calories

LUNCH

Food Item	Serving Size	Carbs	Fats	Protein	Calories

DINNER

Food Item	Serving Size	Carbs	Fats	Protein	Calories

SNACK

Food Item	Serving Size	Carbs	Fats	Protein	Protein

		Carbs	Fats	Protein	Calories
Total For The Day					

Glasses of Water:
☐ ☐ ☐ ☐ ☐ ☐ ☐ ☐ ☐ ☐ ☐ ☐

				Comments
Supplement Intake:	Yes: ☐	No: ☐		
Electrolyte Intake:	Yes: ☐	No: ☐		
In Ketosis:	Yes: ☐	No: ☐		
Exercise:	Yes: ☐	No: ☐		

.... Day.....................Month.......................Year   M T W T F S Sun
☐ ☐ ☐ ☐ ☐ ☐ ☐

BREAKFAST

Food Item	Serving Size	Carbs	Fats	Protein	Calories

LUNCH

Food Item	Serving Size	Carbs	Fats	Protein	Calories

DINNER

Food Item	Serving Size	Carbs	Fats	Protein	Calories

SNACK

Food Item	Serving Size	Carbs	Fats	Protein	Protein

		Carbs	Fats	Protein	Calories
Total For The Day					

Glasses of Water:

☐ ☐ ☐ ☐ ☐ ☐ ☐ ☐ ☐ ☐ ☐ ☐ ☐

Comments

Supplement Intake:	Yes: ☐	No: ☐
Electrolyte Intake:	Yes: ☐	No: ☐
In Ketosis:	Yes: ☐	No: ☐
Exercise:	Yes: ☐	No: ☐

.... Day....................Month......................Year

M T W T F S Sun
☐ ☐ ☐ ☐ ☐ ☐ ☐

BREAKFAST

Food Item	Serving Size	Carbs	Fats	Protein	Calories

LUNCH

Food Item	Serving Size	Carbs	Fats	Protein	Calories

DINNER

Food Item	Serving Size	Carbs	Fats	Protein	Calories

SNACK

Food Item	Serving Size	Carbs	Fats	Protein	Protein

		Carbs	Fats	Protein	Calories
Total For The Day					

Glasses of Water:

☐ ☐ ☐ ☐ ☐ ☐ ☐ ☐ ☐ ☐ ☐ ☐

Comments

Supplement Intake:	Yes: ☐	No: ☐
Electrolyte Intake:	Yes: ☐	No: ☐
In Ketosis:	Yes: ☐	No: ☐
Exercise:	Yes: ☐	No: ☐

.... Day.....................Month.....................Year

M T W T F S Sun
☐ ☐ ☐ ☐ ☐ ☐ ☐

BREAKFAST

Food Item	Serving Size	Carbs	Fats	Protein	Calories

LUNCH

Food Item	Serving Size	Carbs	Fats	Protein	Calories

DINNER

Food Item	Serving Size	Carbs	Fats	Protein	Calories

SNACK

Food Item	Serving Size	Carbs	Fats	Protein	Protein

		Carbs	Fats	Protein	Calories
Total For The Day					

Glasses of Water:

☐ ☐ ☐ ☐ ☐ ☐ ☐ ☐ ☐ ☐ ☐ ☐ ☐

Supplement Intake:	Yes: ☐	No: ☐
Electrolyte Intake:	Yes: ☐	No: ☐
In Ketosis:	Yes: ☐	No: ☐
Exercise:	Yes: ☐	No: ☐

Comments

.... Day......................Month......................Year

M T W T F S Sun
☐ ☐ ☐ ☐ ☐ ☐ ☐

BREAKFAST

Food Item	Serving Size	Carbs	Fats	Protein	Calories

LUNCH

Food Item	Serving Size	Carbs	Fats	Protein	Calories

DINNER

Food Item	Serving Size	Carbs	Fats	Protein	Calories

SNACK

Food Item	Serving Size	Carbs	Fats	Protein	Protein

Total For The Day		Carbs	Fats	Protein	Calories

Glasses of Water:	Comments
☐ ☐ ☐ ☐ ☐ ☐ ☐ ☐ ☐ ☐ ☐ ☐	
Supplement Intake: Yes: ☐ No: ☐	
Electrolyte Intake: Yes: ☐ No: ☐	
In Ketosis: Yes: ☐ No: ☐	
Exercise: Yes: ☐ No: ☐	

.... Day.....................Month.......................Year

M T W T F S Sun
☐ ☐ ☐ ☐ ☐ ☐ ☐

BREAKFAST

Food Item	Serving Size	Carbs	Fats	Protein	Calories

LUNCH

Food Item	Serving Size	Carbs	Fats	Protein	Calories

DINNER

Food Item	Serving Size	Carbs	Fats	Protein	Calories

SNACK

Food Item	Serving Size	Carbs	Fats	Protein	Protein

		Carbs	Fats	Protein	Calories
Total For The Day					

Glasses of Water:

☐ ☐ ☐ ☐ ☐ ☐ ☐ ☐ ☐ ☐ ☐ ☐ ☐

				Comments
Supplement Intake:	Yes: ☐	No: ☐		
Electrolyte Intake:	Yes: ☐	No: ☐		
In Ketosis:	Yes: ☐	No: ☐		
Exercise:	Yes: ☐	No: ☐		

.... Day.....................Month.....................Year

M T W T F S Sun
☐ ☐ ☐ ☐ ☐ ☐ ☐

BREAKFAST

Food Item	Serving Size	Carbs	Fats	Protein	Calories

LUNCH

Food Item	Serving Size	Carbs	Fats	Protein	Calories

DINNER

Food Item	Serving Size	Carbs	Fats	Protein	Calories

SNACK

Food Item	Serving Size	Carbs	Fats	Protein	Protein

		Carbs	Fats	Protein	Calories
Total For The Day					

Glasses of Water:

☐ ☐ ☐ ☐ ☐ ☐ ☐ ☐ ☐ ☐ ☐ ☐

Comments

Supplement Intake:	Yes: ☐	No: ☐
Electrolyte Intake:	Yes: ☐	No: ☐
In Ketosis:	Yes: ☐	No: ☐
Exercise:	Yes: ☐	No: ☐

.... Day.....................Month.......................Year

M T W T F S Sun
□ □ □ □ □ □ □

BREAKFAST

Food Item	Serving Size	Carbs	Fats	Protein	Calories

LUNCH

Food Item	Serving Size	Carbs	Fats	Protein	Calories

DINNER

Food Item	Serving Size	Carbs	Fats	Protein	Calories

SNACK

Food Item	Serving Size	Carbs	Fats	Protein	Protein

		Carbs	Fats	Protein	Calories
Total For The Day					

Glasses of Water:
□ □ □ □ □ □ □ □ □ □ □ □ □ □

Comments

Supplement Intake:	Yes: ☐	No: ☐	
Electrolyte Intake:	Yes: ☐	No: ☐	
In Ketosis:	Yes: ☐	No: ☐	
Exercise:	Yes: ☐	No: ☐	

.... Day.....................Month.....................Year

M T W T F S Sun
□ □ □ □ □ □ □

BREAKFAST

Food Item	Serving Size	Carbs	Fats	Protein	Calories

LUNCH

Food Item	Serving Size	Carbs	Fats	Protein	Calories

DINNER

Food Item	Serving Size	Carbs	Fats	Protein	Calories

SNACK

Food Item	Serving Size	Carbs	Fats	Protein	Protein

		Carbs	Fats	Protein	Calories
Total For The Day					

Glasses of Water:
□ □ □ □ □ □ □ □ □ □ □ □ □

Supplement Intake:	Yes: ☐	No: ☐	
Electrolyte Intake:	Yes: ☐	No: ☐	
In Ketosis:	Yes: ☐	No: ☐	
Exercise:	Yes: ☐	No: ☐	

Comments

.... Day.....................Month.....................Year

M T W T F S Sun
☐ ☐ ☐ ☐ ☐ ☐ ☐

BREAKFAST

Food Item	Serving Size	Carbs	Fats	Protein	Calories

LUNCH

Food Item	Serving Size	Carbs	Fats	Protein	Calories

DINNER

Food Item	Serving Size	Carbs	Fats	Protein	Calories

SNACK

Food Item	Serving Size	Carbs	Fats	Protein	Protein

		Carbs	Fats	Protein	Calories
Total For The Day					

Glasses of Water:	Comments
☐ ☐ ☐ ☐ ☐ ☐ ☐ ☐ ☐ ☐ ☐ ☐ ☐	

Supplement Intake:	Yes: ☐	No: ☐	
Electrolyte Intake:	Yes: ☐	No: ☐	
In Ketosis:	Yes: ☐	No: ☐	
Exercise:	Yes: ☐	No: ☐	

.... Day.....................Month.....................Year

M T W T F S Sun
☐ ☐ ☐ ☐ ☐ ☐ ☐

BREAKFAST

Food Item	Serving Size	Carbs	Fats	Protein	Calories

LUNCH

Food Item	Serving Size	Carbs	Fats	Protein	Calories

DINNER

Food Item	Serving Size	Carbs	Fats	Protein	Calories

SNACK

Food Item	Serving Size	Carbs	Fats	Protein	Protein

		Carbs	Fats	Protein	Calories
Total For The Day					

Glasses of Water:

☐ ☐ ☐ ☐ ☐ ☐ ☐ ☐ ☐ ☐ ☐ ☐ ☐

Supplement Intake:	Yes: ☐	No: ☐
Electrolyte Intake:	Yes: ☐	No: ☐
In Ketosis:	Yes: ☐	No: ☐
Exercise:	Yes: ☐	No: ☐

Comments

.... Day.....................Month.....................Year

M T W T F S Sun
□ □ □ □ □ □ □

BREAKFAST

Food Item	Serving Size	Carbs	Fats	Protein	Calories

LUNCH

Food Item	Serving Size	Carbs	Fats	Protein	Calories

DINNER

Food Item	Serving Size	Carbs	Fats	Protein	Calories

SNACK

Food Item	Serving Size	Carbs	Fats	Protein	Protein

		Carbs	Fats	Protein	Calories
Total For The Day					

Glasses of Water:
□ □ □ □ □ □ □ □ □ □ □ □ □

Comments

Supplement Intake:	Yes: ☐	No: ☐
Electrolyte Intake:	Yes: ☐	No: ☐
In Ketosis:	Yes: ☐	No: ☐
Exercise:	Yes: ☐	No: ☐

.... Day.....................Month.....................Year

M T W T F S Sun
☐ ☐ ☐ ☐ ☐ ☐ ☐

BREAKFAST

Food Item	Serving Size	Carbs	Fats	Protein	Calories

LUNCH

Food Item	Serving Size	Carbs	Fats	Protein	Calories

DINNER

Food Item	Serving Size	Carbs	Fats	Protein	Calories

SNACK

Food Item	Serving Size	Carbs	Fats	Protein	Protein

		Carbs	Fats	Protein	Calories
Total For The Day					

Glasses of Water:

☐ ☐ ☐ ☐ ☐ ☐ ☐ ☐ ☐ ☐ ☐ ☐ ☐

Supplement Intake:	Yes: ☐	No: ☐
Electrolyte Intake:	Yes: ☐	No: ☐
In Ketosis:	Yes: ☐	No: ☐
Exercise:	Yes: ☐	No: ☐

Comments

.... Day.....................Month.......................Year

M T W T F S Sun
☐ ☐ ☐ ☐ ☐ ☐ ☐

BREAKFAST

Food Item	Serving Size	Carbs	Fats	Protein	Calories

LUNCH

Food Item	Serving Size	Carbs	Fats	Protein	Calories

DINNER

Food Item	Serving Size	Carbs	Fats	Protein	Calories

SNACK

Food Item	Serving Size	Carbs	Fats	Protein	Protein

		Carbs	Fats	Protein	Calories
Total For The Day					

Glasses of Water:

☐ ☐ ☐ ☐ ☐ ☐ ☐ ☐ ☐ ☐ ☐ ☐ ☐ ☐

Supplement Intake:	Yes: ☐	No: ☐
Electrolyte Intake:	Yes: ☐	No: ☐
In Ketosis:	Yes: ☐	No: ☐
Exercise:	Yes: ☐	No: ☐

Comments

.... Day.......................Month.......................Year

M T W T F S Sun
☐ ☐ ☐ ☐ ☐ ☐ ☐

BREAKFAST

Food Item	Serving Size	Carbs	Fats	Protein	Calories

LUNCH

Food Item	Serving Size	Carbs	Fats	Protein	Calories

DINNER

Food Item	Serving Size	Carbs	Fats	Protein	Calories

SNACK

Food Item	Serving Size	Carbs	Fats	Protein	Protein

		Carbs	Fats	Protein	Calories
Total For The Day					

Glasses of Water:

☐ ☐ ☐ ☐ ☐ ☐ ☐ ☐ ☐ ☐ ☐ ☐

				Comments
Supplement Intake:	Yes: ☐	No: ☐		
Electrolyte Intake:	Yes: ☐	No: ☐		
In Ketosis:	Yes: ☐	No: ☐		
Exercise:	Yes: ☐	No: ☐		

.... Day.....................Month.....................Year

M T W T F S Sun
□ □ □ □ □ □ □

BREAKFAST

Food Item	Serving Size	Carbs	Fats	Protein	Calories

LUNCH

Food Item	Serving Size	Carbs	Fats	Protein	Calories

DINNER

Food Item	Serving Size	Carbs	Fats	Protein	Calories

SNACK

Food Item	Serving Size	Carbs	Fats	Protein	Protein

Total For The Day		Carbs	Fats	Protein	Calories

Glasses of Water:
□ □ □ □ □ □ □ □ □ □ □ □ □

Supplement Intake:	Yes: ☐	No: ☐
Electrolyte Intake:	Yes: ☐	No: ☐
In Ketosis:	Yes: ☐	No: ☐
Exercise:	Yes: ☐	No: ☐

Comments

.... Day.....................Month.......................Year

M T W T F S Sun
☐ ☐ ☐ ☐ ☐ ☐ ☐

BREAKFAST

Food Item	Serving Size	Carbs	Fats	Protein	Calories

LUNCH

Food Item	Serving Size	Carbs	Fats	Protein	Calories

DINNER

Food Item	Serving Size	Carbs	Fats	Protein	Calories

SNACK

Food Item	Serving Size	Carbs	Fats	Protein	Protein

Total For The Day		Carbs	Fats	Protein	Calories

Glasses of Water:

☐ ☐ ☐ ☐ ☐ ☐ ☐ ☐ ☐ ☐ ☐ ☐ ☐

Comments

Supplement Intake:	Yes: ☐	No: ☐
Electrolyte Intake:	Yes: ☐	No: ☐
In Ketosis:	Yes: ☐	No: ☐
Exercise:	Yes: ☐	No: ☐

.... Day.....................Month.....................Year

M T W T F S Sun
☐ ☐ ☐ ☐ ☐ ☐ ☐

BREAKFAST

Food Item	Serving Size	Carbs	Fats	Protein	Calories

LUNCH

Food Item	Serving Size	Carbs	Fats	Protein	Calories

DINNER

Food Item	Serving Size	Carbs	Fats	Protein	Calories

SNACK

Food Item	Serving Size	Carbs	Fats	Protein	Protein

		Carbs	Fats	Protein	Calories
Total For The Day					

Glasses of Water:

☐ ☐ ☐ ☐ ☐ ☐ ☐ ☐ ☐ ☐ ☐ ☐ ☐ ☐

Comments

Supplement Intake:	Yes: ☐	No: ☐	
Electrolyte Intake:	Yes: ☐	No: ☐	
In Ketosis:	Yes: ☐	No: ☐	
Exercise:	Yes: ☐	No: ☐	

.... Day.....................Month.......................Year

M T W T F S Sun
☐ ☐ ☐ ☐ ☐ ☐ ☐

BREAKFAST

Food Item	Serving Size	Carbs	Fats	Protein	Calories

LUNCH

Food Item	Serving Size	Carbs	Fats	Protein	Calories

DINNER

Food Item	Serving Size	Carbs	Fats	Protein	Calories

SNACK

Food Item	Serving Size	Carbs	Fats	Protein	Protein

		Carbs	Fats	Protein	Calories
Total For The Day					

Glasses of Water:	Comments
☐ ☐ ☐ ☐ ☐ ☐ ☐ ☐ ☐ ☐ ☐ ☐	

Supplement Intake:	Yes: ☐	No: ☐		
Electrolyte Intake:	Yes: ☐	No: ☐		
In Ketosis:	Yes: ☐	No: ☐		
Exercise:	Yes: ☐	No: ☐		

.... Day.....................Month.....................Year

M T W T F S Sun
☐ ☐ ☐ ☐ ☐ ☐ ☐

BREAKFAST

Food Item	Serving Size	Carbs	Fats	Protein	Calories

LUNCH

Food Item	Serving Size	Carbs	Fats	Protein	Calories

DINNER

Food Item	Serving Size	Carbs	Fats	Protein	Calories

SNACK

Food Item	Serving Size	Carbs	Fats	Protein	Protein

		Carbs	Fats	Protein	Calories
Total For The Day					

Glasses of Water:

☐ ☐ ☐ ☐ ☐ ☐ ☐ ☐ ☐ ☐ ☐ ☐

Comments

Supplement Intake:	Yes: ☐	No: ☐
Electrolyte Intake:	Yes: ☐	No: ☐
In Ketosis:	Yes: ☐	No: ☐
Exercise:	Yes: ☐	No: ☐

.... Day......................Month......................Year

M T W T F S Sun
☐ ☐ ☐ ☐ ☐ ☐ ☐

BREAKFAST

Food Item	Serving Size	Carbs	Fats	Protein	Calories

LUNCH

Food Item	Serving Size	Carbs	Fats	Protein	Calories

DINNER

Food Item	Serving Size	Carbs	Fats	Protein	Calories

SNACK

Food Item	Serving Size	Carbs	Fats	Protein	Protein

		Carbs	Fats	Protein	Calories
Total For The Day					

Glasses of Water:
☐ ☐ ☐ ☐ ☐ ☐ ☐ ☐ ☐ ☐ ☐ ☐ ☐

Supplement Intake:	Yes: ☐	No: ☐
Electrolyte Intake:	Yes: ☐	No: ☐
In Ketosis:	Yes: ☐	No: ☐
Exercise:	Yes: ☐	No: ☐

Comments

.... Day.....................Month.....................Year

M T W T F S Sun
□ □ □ □ □ □ □

BREAKFAST

Food Item	Serving Size	Carbs	Fats	Protein	Calories

LUNCH

Food Item	Serving Size	Carbs	Fats	Protein	Calories

DINNER

Food Item	Serving Size	Carbs	Fats	Protein	Calories

SNACK

Food Item	Serving Size	Carbs	Fats	Protein	Protein

Total For The Day		Carbs	Fats	Protein	Calories

Glasses of Water:
□ □ □ □ □ □ □ □ □ □ □ □ □

Comments

Supplement Intake:	Yes: ☐	No: ☐
Electrolyte Intake:	Yes: ☐	No: ☐
In Ketosis:	Yes: ☐	No: ☐
Exercise:	Yes: ☐	No: ☐

.... Day.....................Month.....................Year

M T W T F S Sun
☐ ☐ ☐ ☐ ☐ ☐ ☐

BREAKFAST

Food Item	Serving Size	Carbs	Fats	Protein	Calories

LUNCH

Food Item	Serving Size	Carbs	Fats	Protein	Calories

DINNER

Food Item	Serving Size	Carbs	Fats	Protein	Calories

SNACK

Food Item	Serving Size	Carbs	Fats	Protein	Protein

		Carbs	Fats	Protein	Calories
Total For The Day					

Glasses of Water:
☐ ☐ ☐ ☐ ☐ ☐ ☐ ☐ ☐ ☐ ☐ ☐

Comments

Supplement Intake:	Yes: ☐	No: ☐
Electrolyte Intake:	Yes: ☐	No: ☐
In Ketosis:	Yes: ☐	No: ☐
Exercise:	Yes: ☐	No: ☐

.... Day.....................Month......................Year

M T W T F S Sun
☐ ☐ ☐ ☐ ☐ ☐ ☐

BREAKFAST

Food Item	Serving Size	Carbs	Fats	Protein	Calories

LUNCH

Food Item	Serving Size	Carbs	Fats	Protein	Calories

DINNER

Food Item	Serving Size	Carbs	Fats	Protein	Calories

SNACK

Food Item	Serving Size	Carbs	Fats	Protein	Protein

		Carbs	Fats	Protein	Calories
Total For The Day					

Glasses of Water:

☐ ☐ ☐ ☐ ☐ ☐ ☐ ☐ ☐ ☐ ☐ ☐ ☐

			Comments
Supplement Intake:	Yes: ☐	No: ☐	
Electrolyte Intake:	Yes: ☐	No: ☐	
In Ketosis:	Yes: ☐	No: ☐	
Exercise:	Yes: ☐	No: ☐	

.... Day.....................Month.....................Year

M T W T F S Sun
☐ ☐ ☐ ☐ ☐ ☐ ☐

BREAKFAST

Food Item	Serving Size	Carbs	Fats	Protein	Calories

LUNCH

Food Item	Serving Size	Carbs	Fats	Protein	Calories

DINNER

Food Item	Serving Size	Carbs	Fats	Protein	Calories

SNACK

Food Item	Serving Size	Carbs	Fats	Protein	Protein

		Carbs	Fats	Protein	Calories
Total For The Day					

Glasses of Water:	Comments
☐ ☐ ☐ ☐ ☐ ☐ ☐ ☐ ☐ ☐ ☐ ☐ ☐	

Supplement Intake: Yes: ☐ No: ☐

Electrolyte Intake: Yes: ☐ No: ☐

In Ketosis: Yes: ☐ No: ☐

Exercise: Yes: ☐ No: ☐

.... Day.......................Month.......................Year

M T W T F S Sun
☐ ☐ ☐ ☐ ☐ ☐ ☐

BREAKFAST

Food Item	Serving Size	Carbs	Fats	Protein	Calories

LUNCH

Food Item	Serving Size	Carbs	Fats	Protein	Calories

DINNER

Food Item	Serving Size	Carbs	Fats	Protein	Calories

SNACK

Food Item	Serving Size	Carbs	Fats	Protein	Protein

		Carbs	Fats	Protein	Calories
Total For The Day					

Glasses of Water:

☐ ☐ ☐ ☐ ☐ ☐ ☐ ☐ ☐ ☐ ☐ ☐ ☐

Comments

Supplement Intake:	Yes: ☐	No: ☐
Electrolyte Intake:	Yes: ☐	No: ☐
In Ketosis:	Yes: ☐	No: ☐
Exercise:	Yes: ☐	No: ☐

.... Day.....................Month......................Year

M T W T F S Sun
☐ ☐ ☐ ☐ ☐ ☐ ☐

BREAKFAST

Food Item	Serving Size	Carbs	Fats	Protein	Calories

LUNCH

Food Item	Serving Size	Carbs	Fats	Protein	Calories

DINNER

Food Item	Serving Size	Carbs	Fats	Protein	Calories

SNACK

Food Item	Serving Size	Carbs	Fats	Protein	Protein

		Carbs	Fats	Protein	Calories
Total For The Day					

Glasses of Water:
☐ ☐ ☐ ☐ ☐ ☐ ☐ ☐ ☐ ☐ ☐ ☐

Comments

Supplement Intake:	Yes: ☐	No: ☐
Electrolyte Intake:	Yes: ☐	No: ☐
In Ketosis:	Yes: ☐	No: ☐
Exercise:	Yes: ☐	No: ☐

WEIGHT LOSS LOG

Start Weight:	
Start Date:	
Weight Goal:	

Date	Weight	+/-

Date	Weight	+/-
Date	Weight	+/-

Date	Weight	+/-
Date	Weight	+/-
Date	Weight	+/-

Date	Weight	+/-
Date	Weight	+/-

Health Report Details

Date	Health Test Name / Indicator Name	Value
	Health Test Name / Indicator Name	

Health Report Details

Date	Health Test Name / Indicator Name	Value
Date	Health Test Name / Indicator Name	Value

Health Report Details

Date	Health Test Name / Indicator Name	Value
Date	Health Test Name / Indicator Name	Value

Health Report Details

Date	Health Test Name / Indicator Name	Value
Date	Health Test Name / Indicator Name	Value

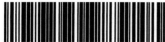

Made in the USA
Middletown, DE
01 August 2018